WATERLOO LOCAL SCHOOL
MIDDLE SCHOOL LIBRARY

An Early Career Book

careers in
BEAUTY & GROOMING

Mark Lerner

photographs by
Milton J. Blumenfeld

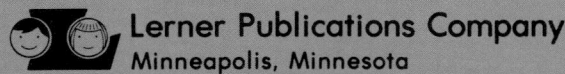
Lerner Publications Company
Minneapolis, Minnesota

LIBRARY OF CONGRESS CATALOGING IN PUBLICATION DATA

Lerner, Mark.
Careers in beauty and grooming.

(An Early Career Book)
SUMMARY: Briefly describes fifteen beauty and grooming careers, such as beauty school instructor, electrologist, product formulation chemist, and beauty salon owner.

1. Beauty culture—Vocational guidance—Juvenile literature. [1. Beauty culture—Vocational guidance. 2. Vocational guidance] I. Blumenfeld, Milton J. II. Title.

TT958.L47   646.7'023   77-72419
ISBN 0-8225-0328-X

Copyright © 1977 by Lerner Publications Company

All rights reserved. International copyright secured. Manufactured in the United States of America. Published simultaneously in Canada by J. M. Dent & Sons (Canada) Ltd., Don Mills, Ontario.

International Standard Book Number: 0-8225-0328-X   Library of Congress Catalog Card Number: 77-72419

1 2 3 4 5 6 7 8 9 10 85 84 83 82 81 80 79 78 77

Would you like to have a career in beauty and grooming?

People in the beauty and grooming field try to help others feel good about the way they look. Most of the people in this field work directly with the *patrons*—those who come to them for service. But some, like chemists, work in places where patrons do not go.

Many of the people who work in the beauty and grooming field must have special training before they can begin their careers. After a person is trained to be a beautician (byoo-TIH-shun) or a barber-hairstylist, he or she must pass special tests given by the state. If the person passes these tests, he or she is given a license and is allowed to work with the public. If you like working with people and making them happy, a career in beauty and grooming may be for you.

BARBER-HAIRSTYLIST

Of all the people in this book, the person you probably know most about is the barber-hairstylist. Barber-hairstylists work on people of all ages. They cut, color, wash, and style hair. And they sometimes give shaves. Barber-hairstylists also show patrons how to take care of their hair. They may suggest a different shampoo or a new hair color. Barber-hairstylists can sell these and other hair care products for use at home.

Barber-hairstylists must go to special schools to be trained for their profession. They must also have licenses from the state before they can work with the public. Some barber-hairstylists work in small one-chair shops. Others work in shops where there are many chairs and many barber-hairstylists.

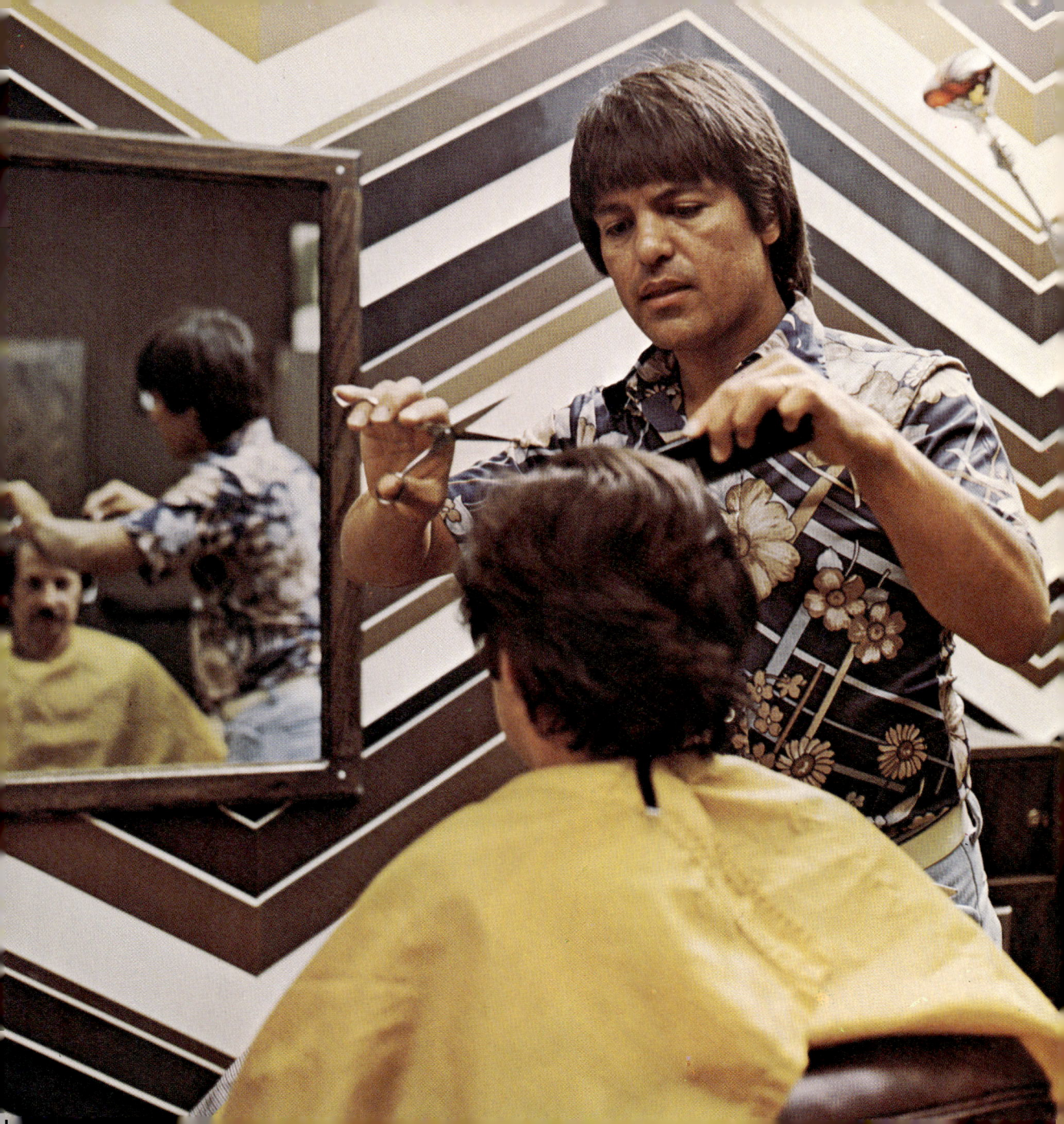

BEAUTICIAN

When a woman wants her hair to look nice for a special occasion, she often visits her beautician. Beauticians are also called hairdressers and cosmetologists (kahz-muh-TAHL-uh-jists). Although beauticians may have men for patrons, most of their patrons are women. Beauticians must go to beauty school and get licenses from the state before they can begin working.

Besides washing, curling, and cutting hair, beauticians can do special things with it. They can give *permanents*. A patron with straight hair, for example, may want curly hair. A beautician can make the hair curly with a permanent. Another special thing that beauticians do is tint hair. In tinting, the color of a patron's hair is changed.

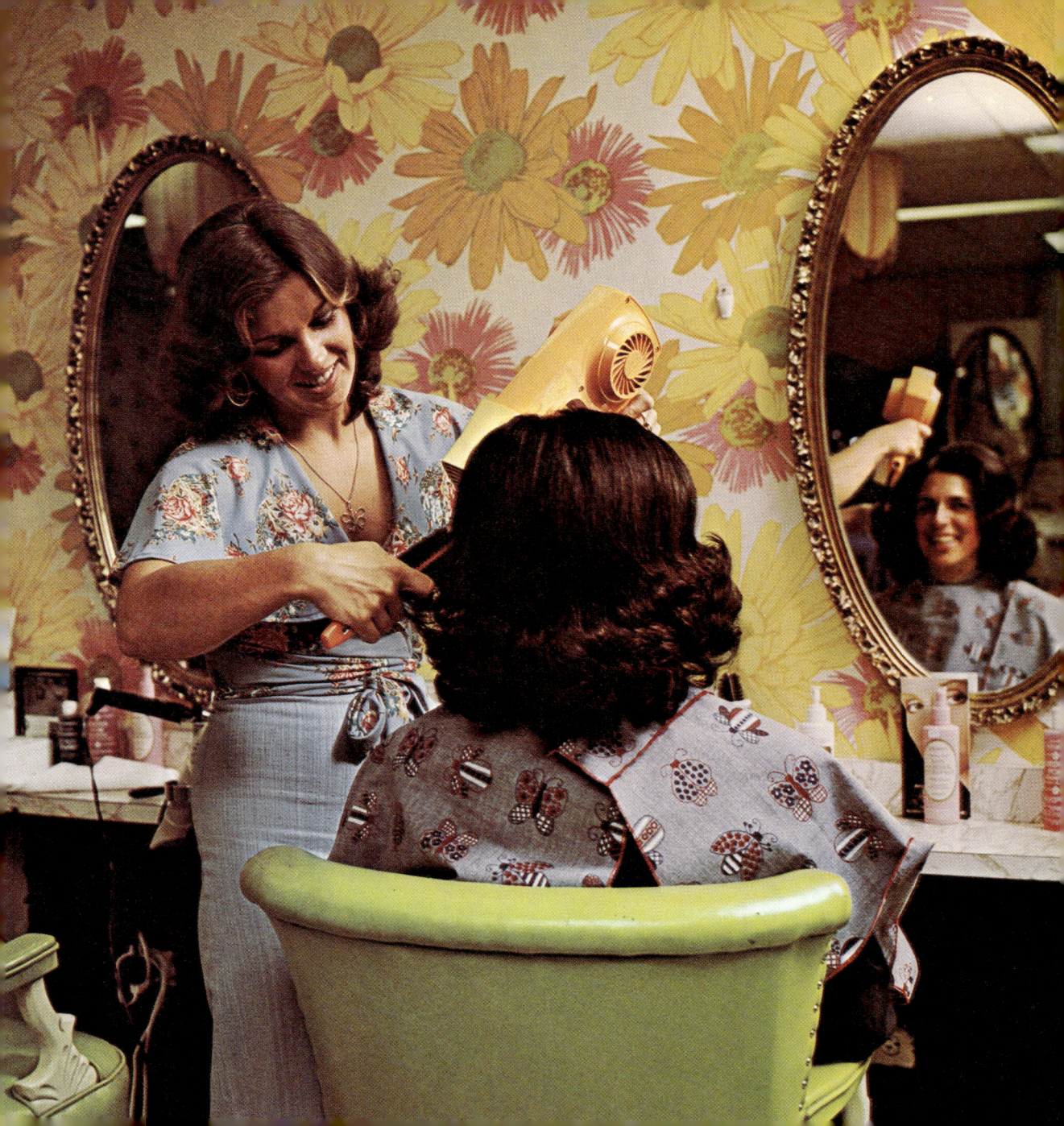

BEAUTICIAN'S ASSISTANT

Beauticians in a salon often need help with their patrons. The beautician's assistant is the beautician's helper. He or she seats patrons and shampoos their hair. While the beautician's assistant is giving one patron a shampoo, the beautician is busy "combing out" another patron. When the beautician and the beautician's assistant work as a team, they can serve many patrons at once.

Some beauticians' assistants are people who have just gotten their licenses to become beauticians. They are anxious to get on-the-job training in a beauty salon. By working in a salon, beauticians' assistants can learn about the finer points of being a beautician. At the same time they can earn money and meet people who may one day become their own patrons.

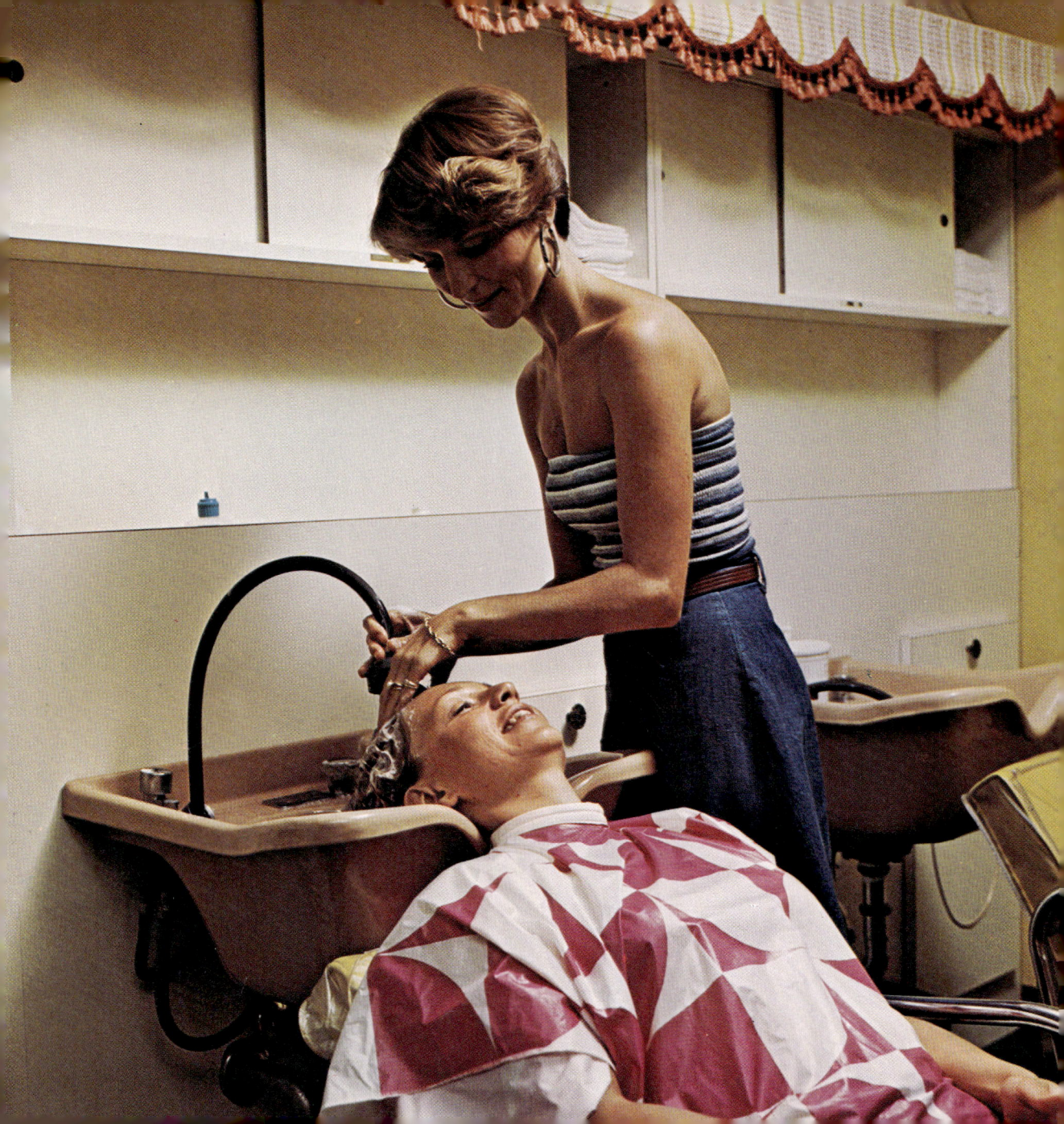

MANICURIST

Manicurists (MAN-ih-cur-ists) take care of their patrons' hands and fingernails. To keep the hands looking nice, manicurists rub lotions on them. Manicurists take old polish off of fingernails or put new polish on, and they use a file to shape the nails nicely. If a patron has a broken or cracked fingernail, the manicurist can mend it. He or she can make a sculptured nail to fit over the injured nail. Sculptured nails are made of a special plastic. Manicurists also work with *cuticles* (KYOO-tih-culs)—the skin at the base of the fingernails. The manicurist not only works on hands and fingernails, but also on feet and toenails. When the manicurist is treating a part of the foot, he or she is giving a *pedicure* (PED-ih-cur).

Manicurists have gone to beauty school to become licensed as beauticians. They also have taken special courses just for manicurists.

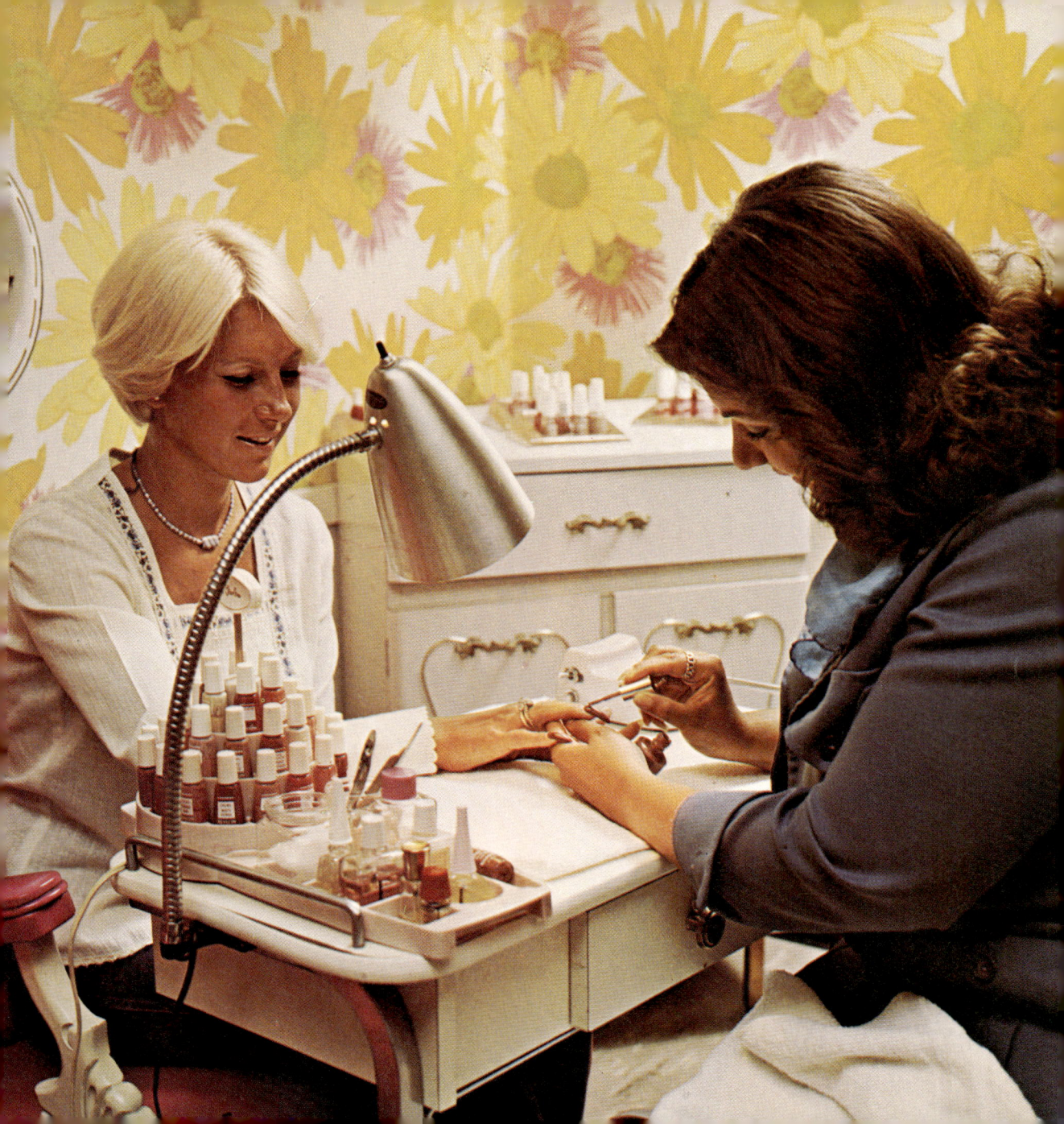

SKIN CARE SPECIALIST

When people want special care for their skin, they sometimes visit skin care specialists. Skin care specialists can take care of dry, oily, or normal skin. If patrons have any skin problems, skin care specialists can suggest products that will help.

To treat the skin on the face, the skin care specialist sometimes gives facials. He or she uses special lotions and creams to do this. Facials help peoples' faces look healthier and feel better. The skin care specialist gives massages, too. To give massages, skin care specialists must know about the muscles, bones, and nerves in a person's body, especially those in the face, neck, and shoulders.

Skin care specialists get their training in beauty school. They are licensed beauticians, but they must have extra training to become skin care specialists.

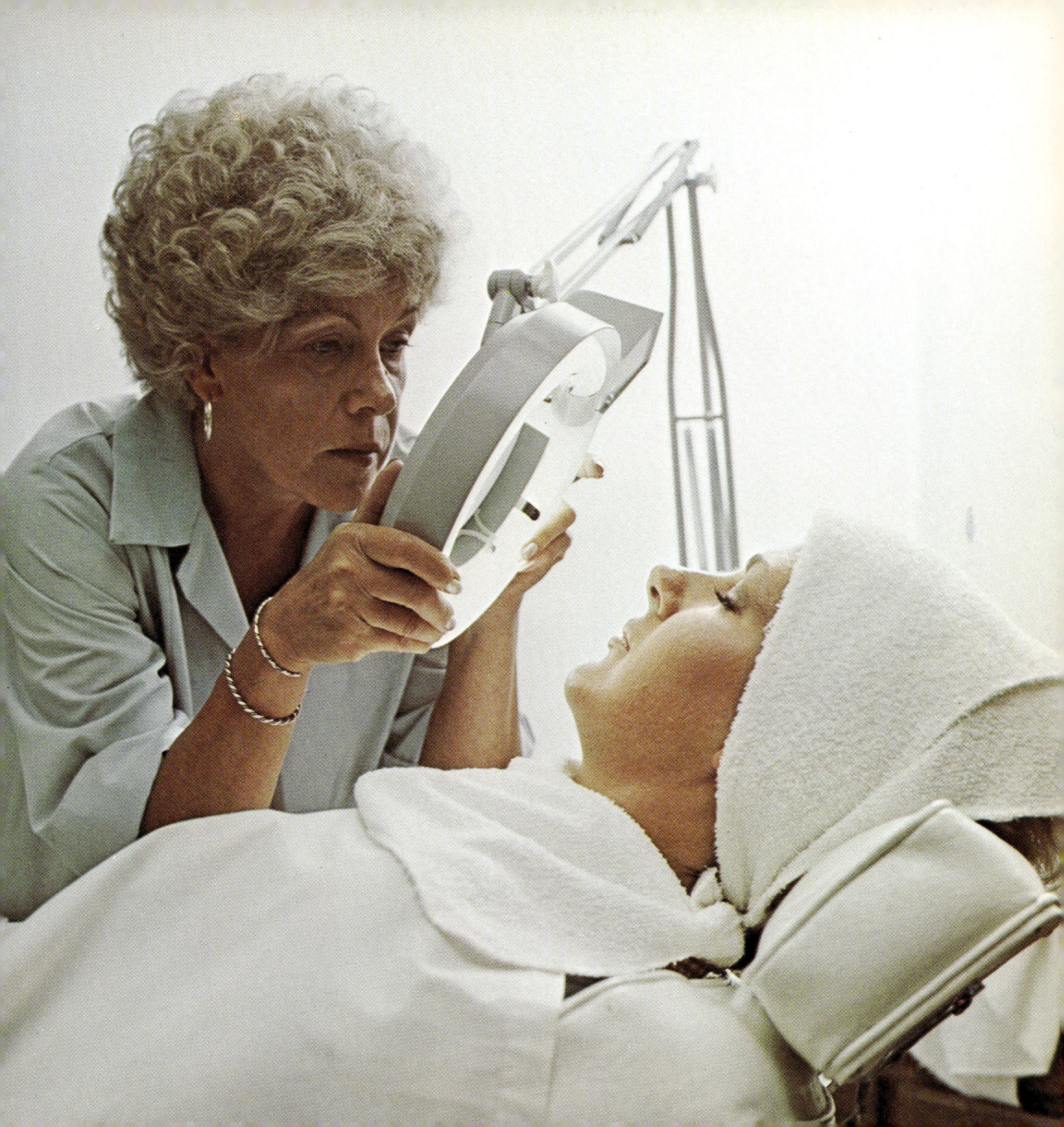

ELECTROLOGIST

When people want to have hair permanently removed from their bodies, they can go to the *electrologist* (eh-lek-TRAHL-uh-jist). The electrologist removes hair from the body by using *electrolysis* (eh-lek-TRAHL-ih-sis). When the electrologist uses electrolysis, he or she puts an electrified needle into the skin where hair is growing. The electric current from the needle kills the hair root so that it will not grow back again. Because electrologists use electricity to burn beneath the skin, they must do their work very carefully. Electrologists must know a lot about hair and the way it grows.

With some people, unwanted hair can cause great problems. Electrologists try to help their patrons overcome these problems by talking with them. Because electrologists know that they are helping people, they get much satisfaction out of the work they do.

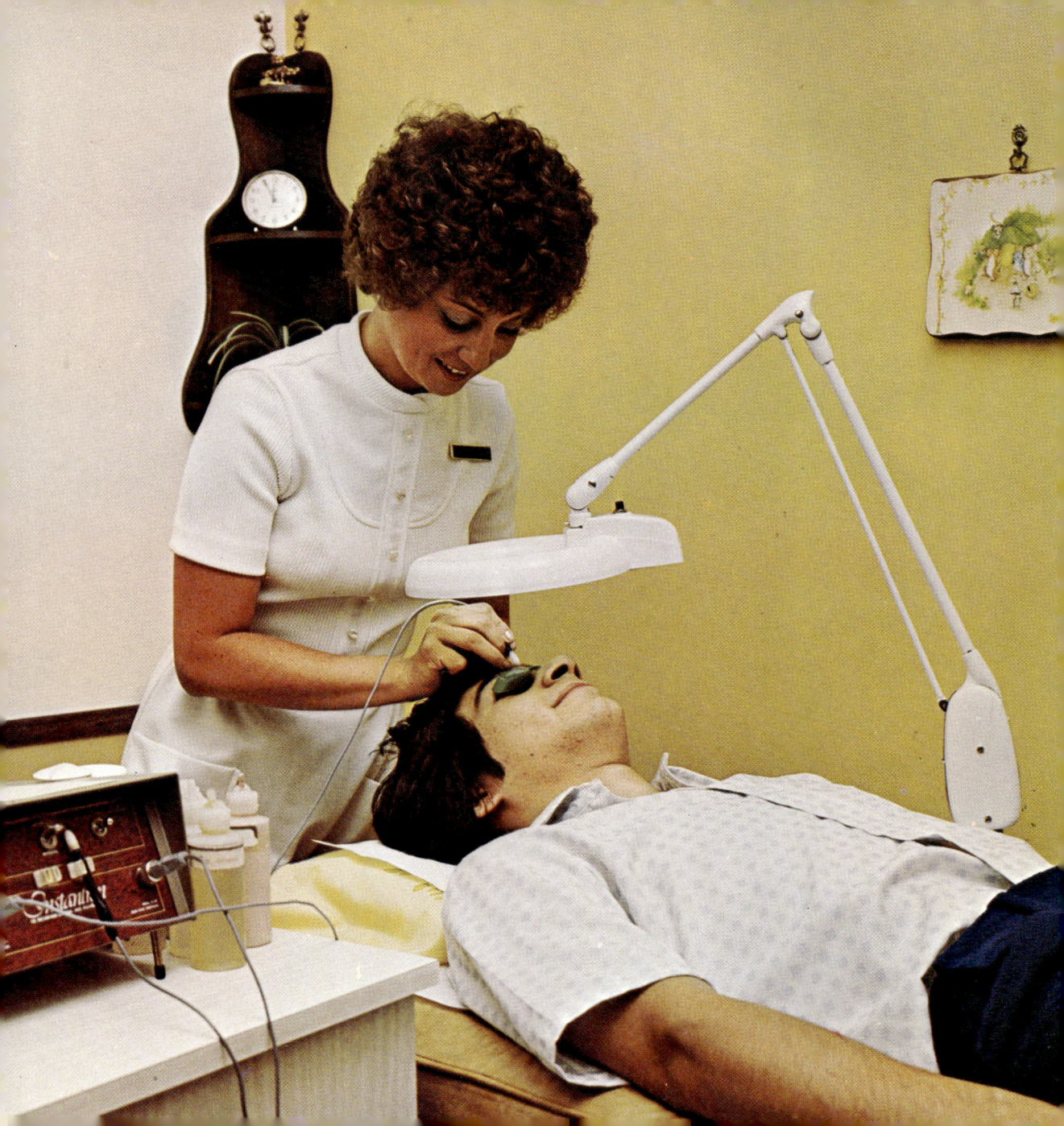

HAIR REPLACEMENT SPECIALIST

Some people lose all or part of their hair—they become *bald*. Baldness happens to men more often than it happens to women. Hair replacement specialists help their bald patrons by fitting them with hairpieces. A hairpiece is human or artificial hair that covers a bald part of the head. Hairpieces are also called *wigs* and *toupees* (too-PAYS).

Not all hairpieces and bald spots are the same size. The hair replacement specialist measures the bald spot on a patron's head. Then he or she decides what kind of hairpiece that person should have. After deciding the size, color, and texture of the hairpiece, the hair replacement specialist orders one from a special company.

Hair replacement specialists also show their patrons how to care for hairpieces. Knowing how to clean and dry a hairpiece is an important part of owning one.

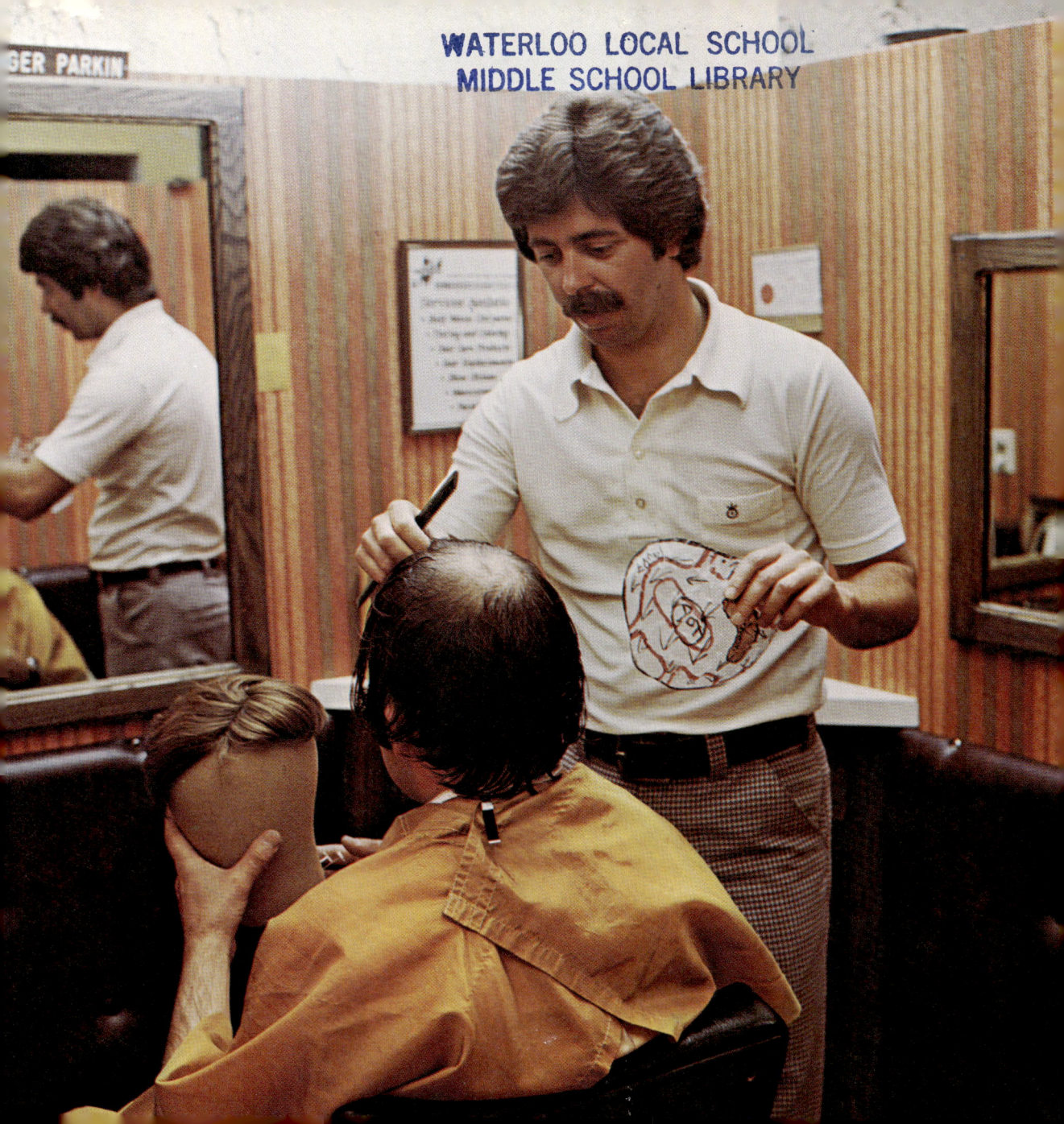

WIG STYLIST

Modern-day wigs are made of both human and synthetic (sin-THET-ik), or artificial, hair. Wig stylists work with both kinds of wigs. They clean, set, cut, and color wigs. They can style wigs in almost any way. Wig stylists must be licensed beauticians before they can become stylists.

Wig stylists work in beauty salons and department stores. When people want to buy wigs, they can ask wig stylists to help them make the right choices. Once in a while, wigs need to be repaired. Wig stylists can also repair wigs. They know how to tighten the elastic that keeps a wig snug. They can also suggest hair care products that will make wigs last longer.

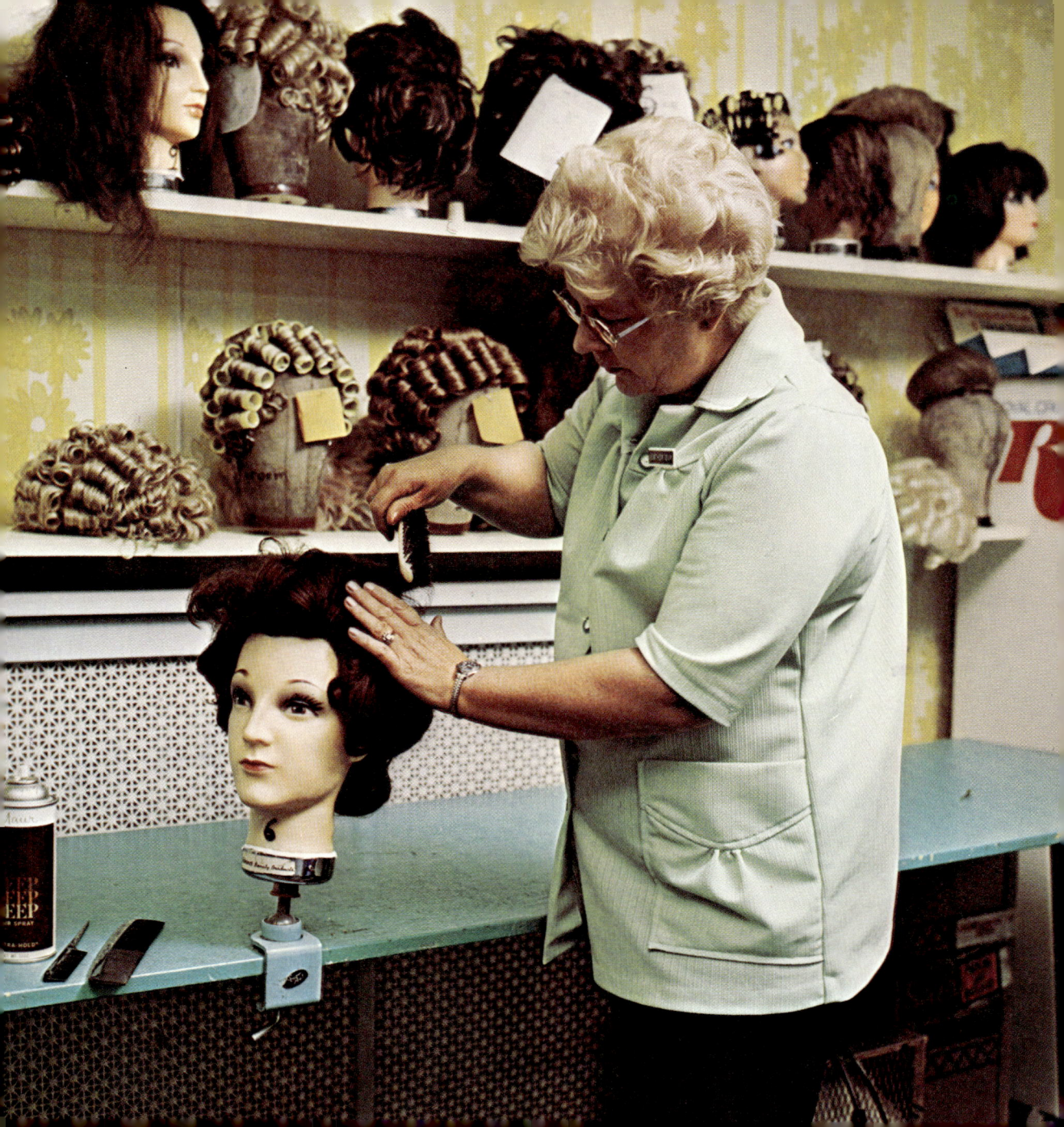

BEAUTY SCHOOL INSTRUCTOR

People need special training to become beauticians. Beauty schools are the places in which people get their training. Beauty school instructors teach students the things they need to know to become qualified beauticians. They teach the many parts of *cosmetology*—the art of beautifying the skin, hair, and nails.

Besides teaching cosmetology, beauty school instructors teach their students other things. They teach health practices, or hygiene (HI-jeen). And they show their students how to work well with many kinds of people. Beauty school instructors give classroom talks and look over their students' work in the practice salon. Patience and a desire to help students learn are two qualities that beauty school instructors must have.

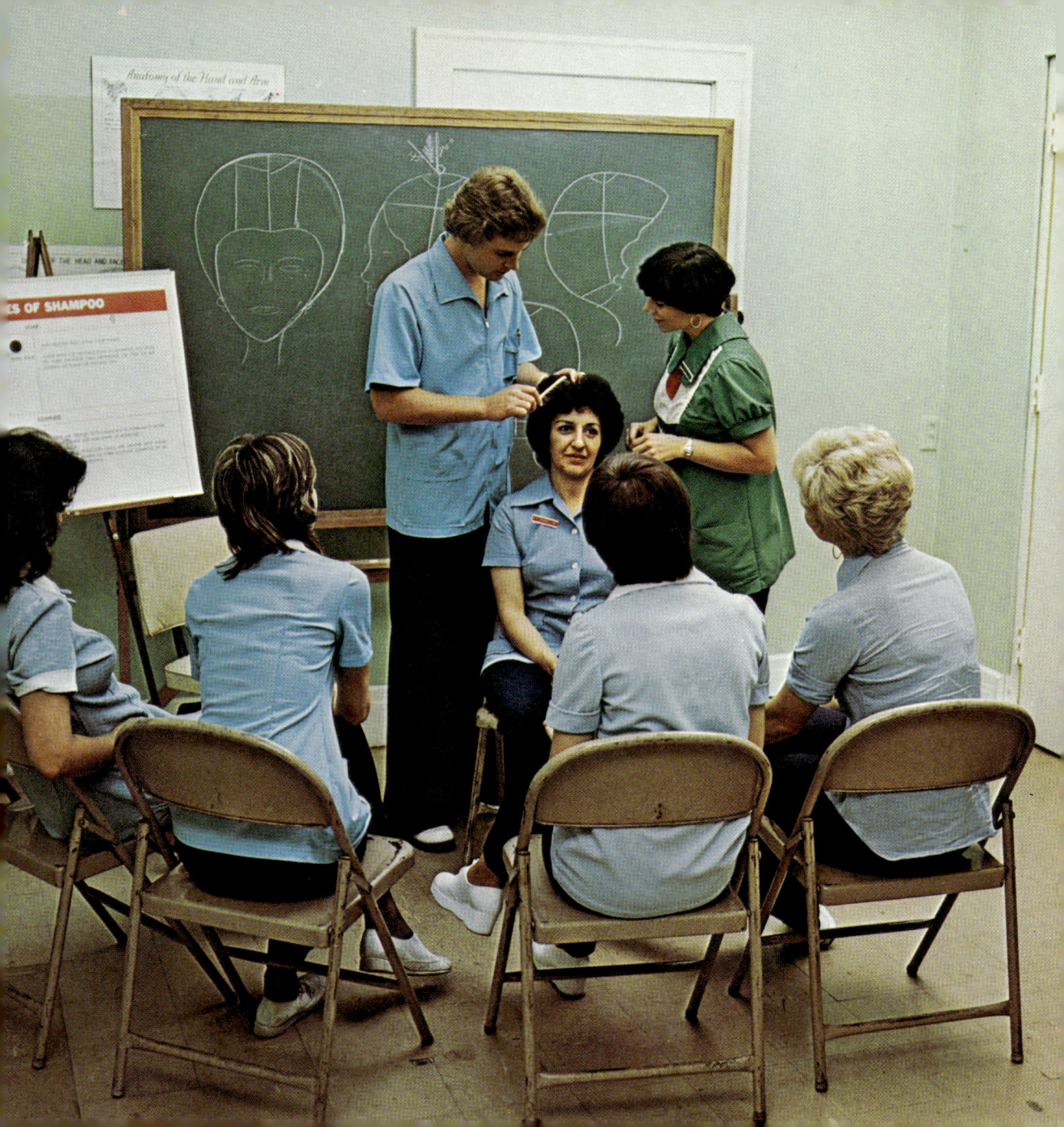

PRODUCT FORMULATION CHEMIST

New cosmetics start out as ideas. In a cosmetics company, ideas for new cosmetics are sent to the product formulation chemist. The product formulation chemist makes new cosmetics from basic ingredients. He or she tests the idea in the laboratory to see whether it can be made into a real product.

After a product has been on the market for a while, the cosmetics company may decide to improve or change some ingredients in it. Product formulation chemists also check the product and try to improve it. They may, for example, add more dye to a hair color, or take away some oil from a skin conditioner.

Product formulation chemists, like most chemists, have been trained for their work in college. In this picture, the product formulation chemist is experimenting with a new liquid makeup.

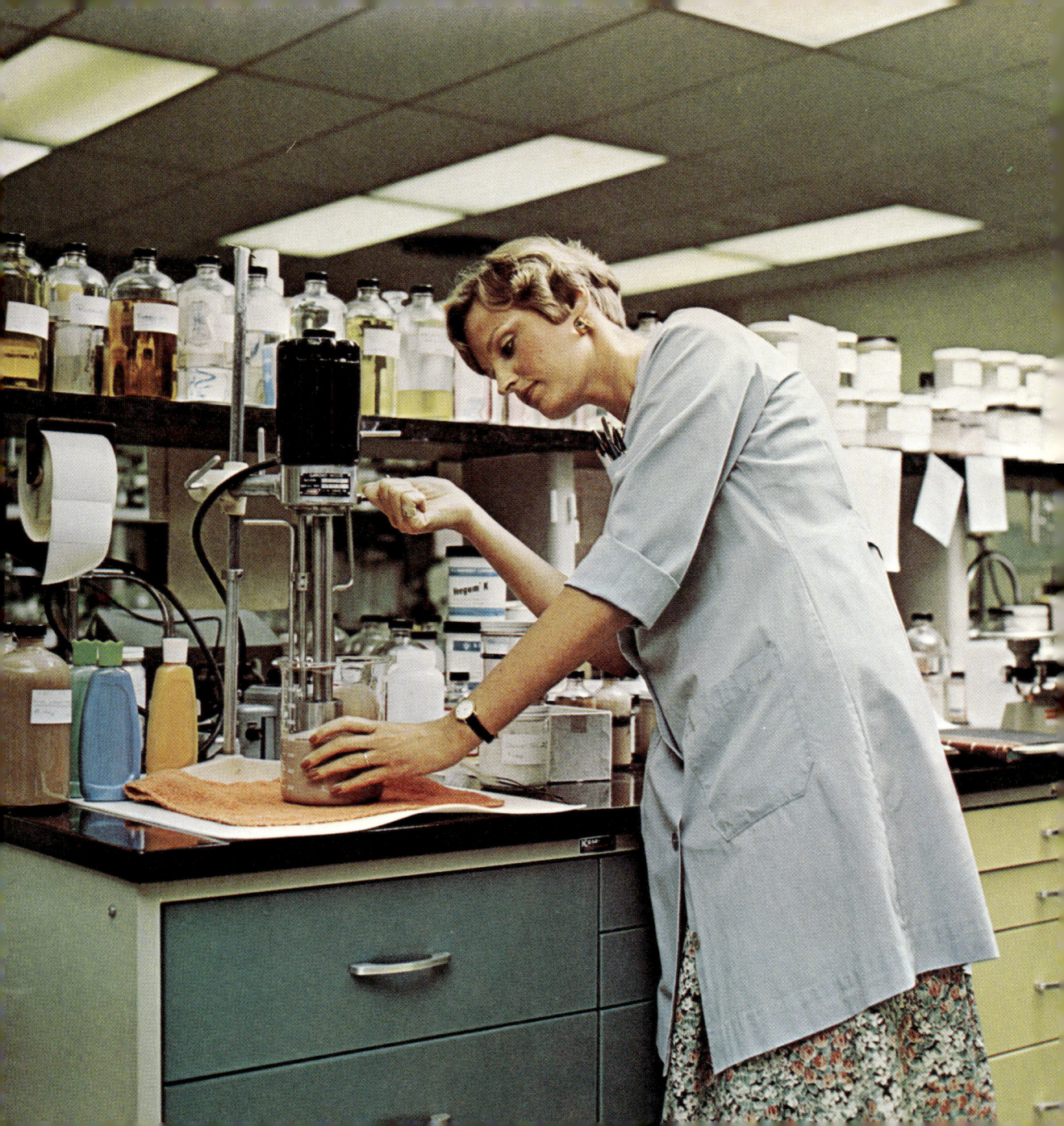

ANALYTICAL RESEARCH CHEMIST

Before a new cosmetic is put on the market, it must meet all health regulations. Analytical research chemists test their companies' cosmetics to make sure that they are safe.

Analytical research chemists also help product formulation chemists with their work. They check the basic ingredients that go into a new cosmetic. And they write down the exact ingredients that go into it, too. This job is called *setting specifications* (spes-ih-fih-KAY-shuns). Specifications must be set to make sure that each time a new batch of a product is made, it will work just as it did before.

Analytical research chemists analyze other companies' products, too. One reason they do this is to learn what special ingredients other companies put into their products.

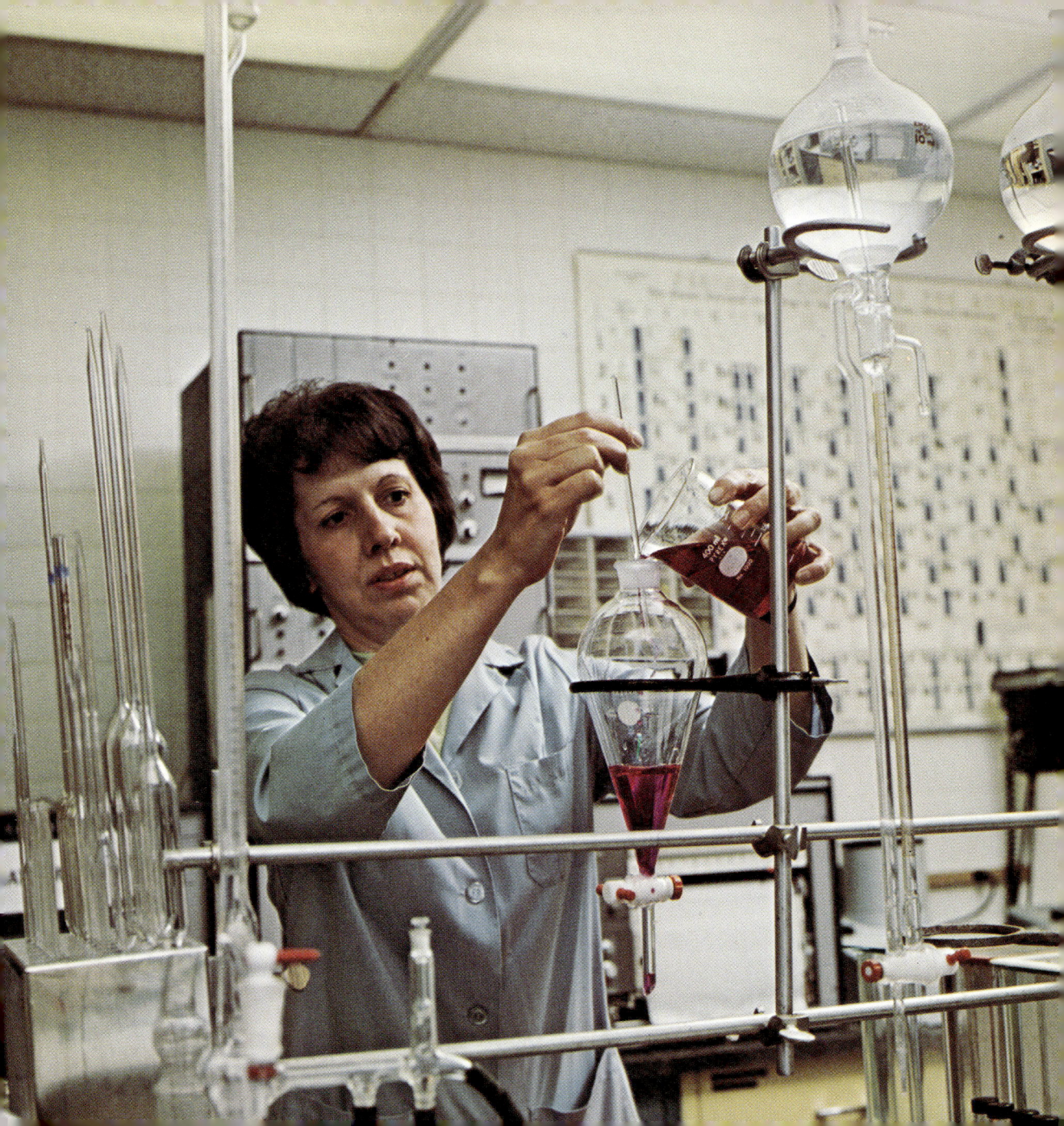

TESTING SALON TECHNICIAN

The testing salon technician is both a chemist and a beautician. He or she tests shampoos and other products on a patron to see how well they work. The testing salon technician will put one kind of shampoo on one side of the patron's head and another shampoo on the other side. By testing two products on the same head, the testing salon technician can decide which one works best. While the testing salon technician is testing the product, he or she is also styling the patron's hair. Patrons are willing to have their hair tested because they get free hair styling done by good beauticians. Testing salon technicians not only test the products made by their own companies, but also those made by other companies.

Testing salon technicians work for companies that make hair products and other cosmetics. They have been to beauty school, and they are licensed beauticians.

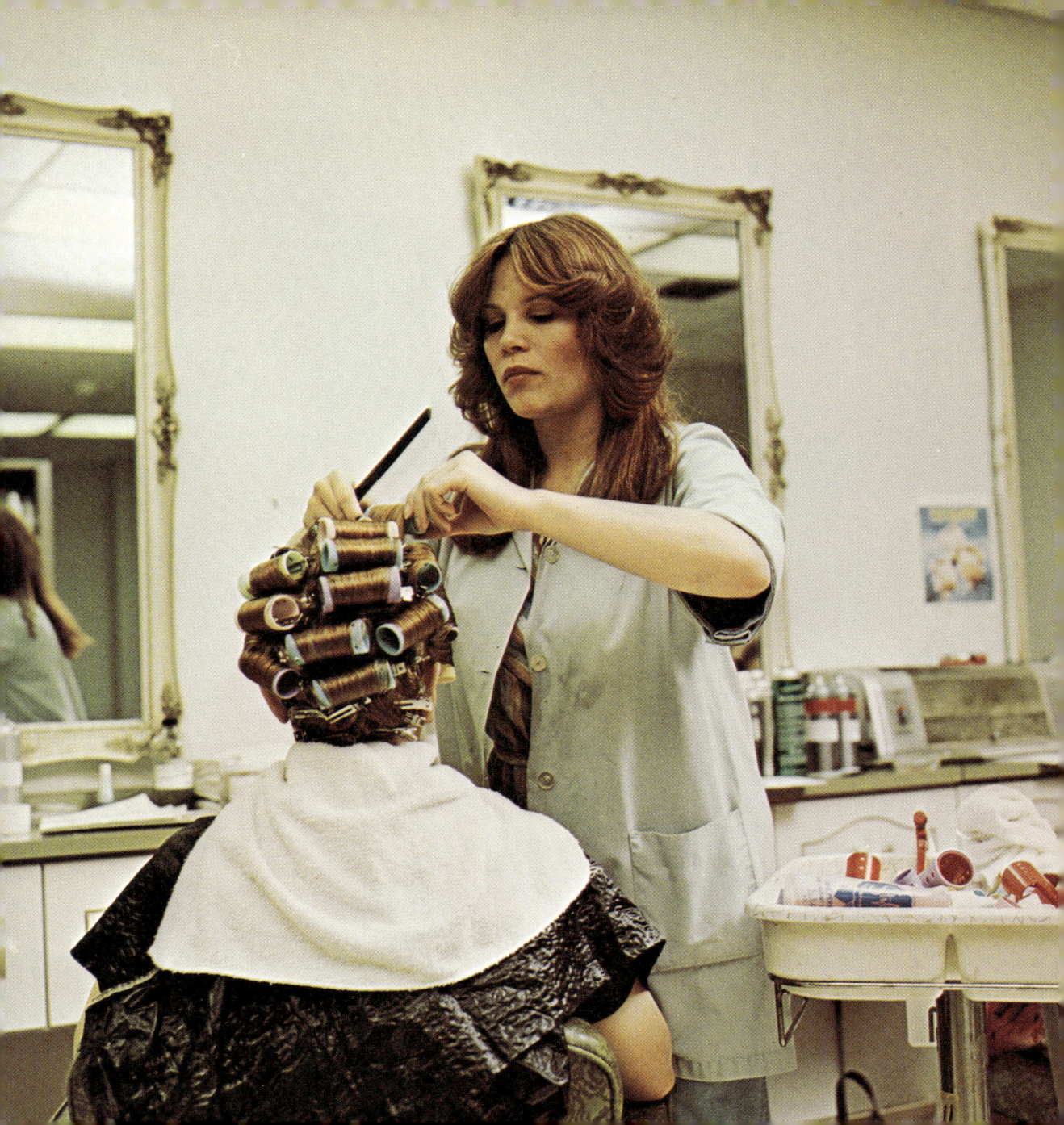

BEAUTY SALON OWNER

Have you ever visited a beauty salon? If you have, you probably noticed the person who greeted you. That cheerful person may have been the beauty salon owner. Besides greeting the patrons, the beauty salon owner talks to people over the telephone. He or she writes down appointments—the time and date that patrons will come to the salon.

All the people who work in the salon, such as the beautician, the manicurist, and the beautician's assistant, are hired by the beauty salon owner. The beauty salon owner also pays for the supplies that are used in the salon. He or she orders more supplies when the salon needs them. Often the beauty salon owner is also a beautician. He or she will sometimes "step behind the chair" and work on special patrons.

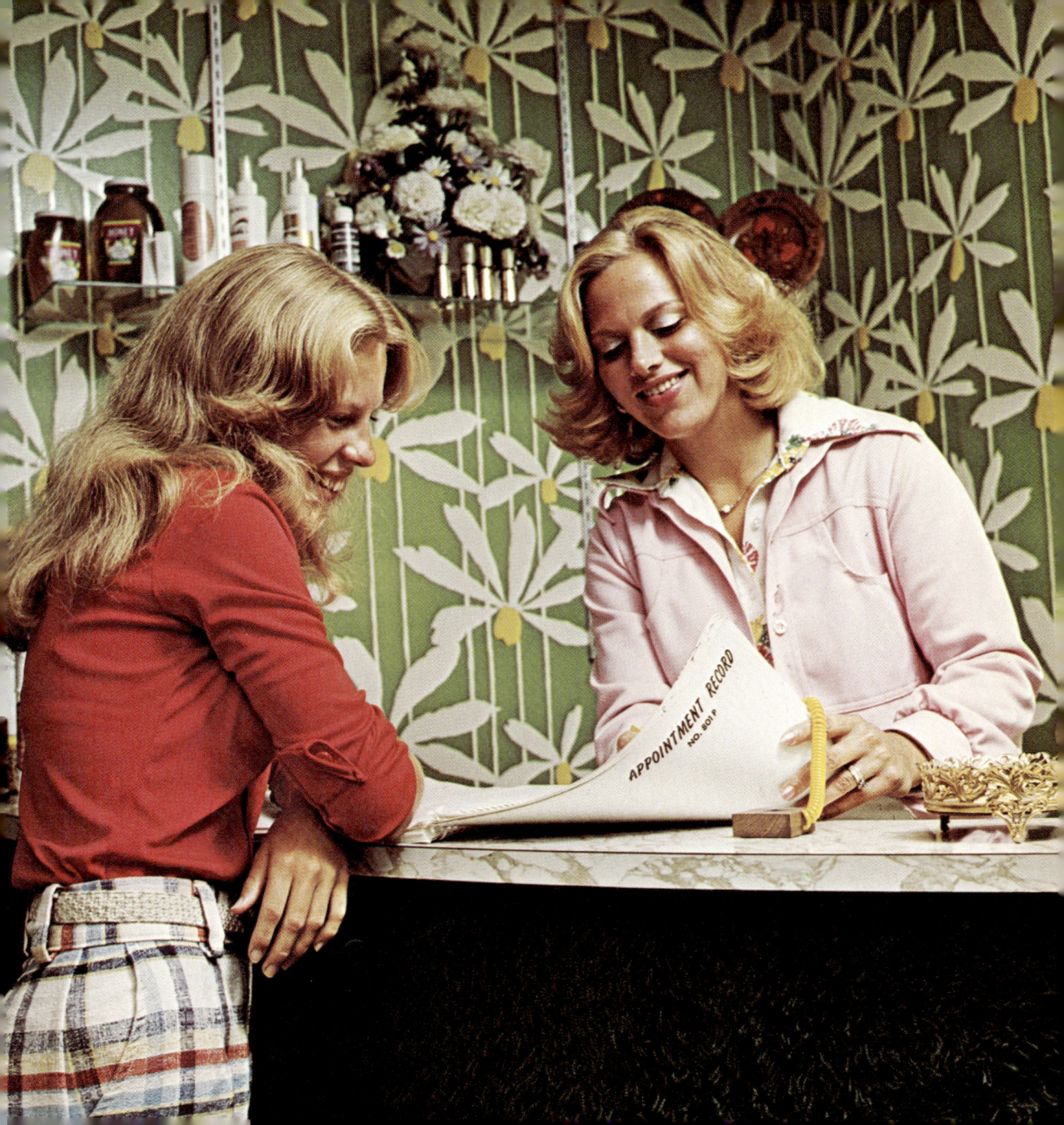

COSMETICS SALESPERSON

Cosmetics salespersons supply beauticians and barber-hairstylists with the products that they need. They sell everything from nail polish to skin cream. Cosmetics salespersons get their products from the cosmetics companies that make them. The cosmetics salespersons give orders to cosmetics companies. And they take orders from beauty salons and barber-hairstylist shops. Because cosmetics salespersons sell to many beauty salons and barber-hairstylist shops, they must keep careful records of the orders that they take. They must also keep careful records of the products that they have ordered from cosmetics companies.

Knowing about the products you sell is an important part of being a cosmetics salesperson.

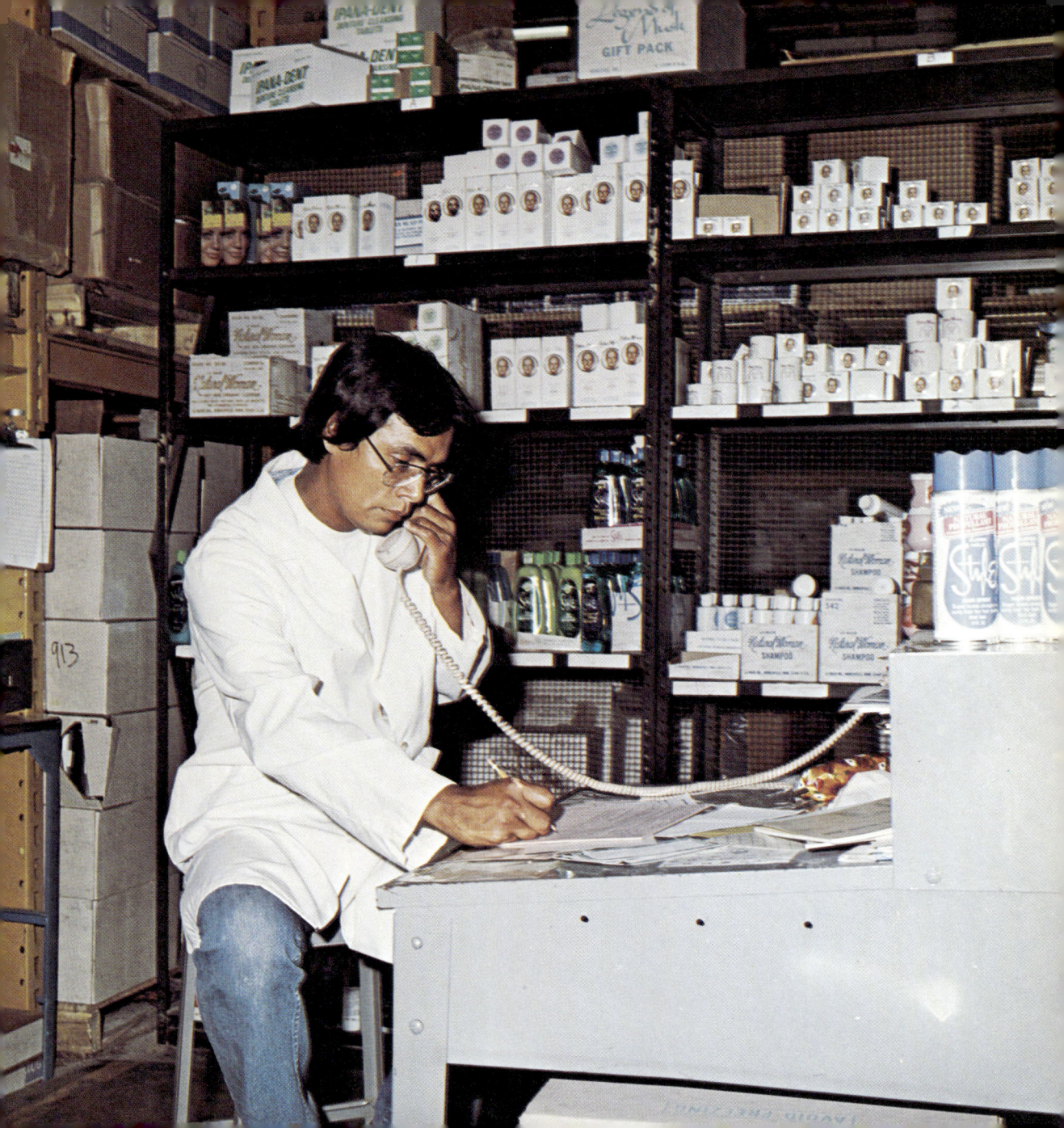

BEAUTY CONSULTANT

Beauty consultants are both teachers and salespersons. They give special parties, or shows, in the homes of people who want to learn about cosmetics and buy them. During the parties, beauty consultants explain to their listeners the best ways to take care of their skin. They show how to put on makeup and how to use many other kinds of cosmetics. Some of the things that beauty consultants sell are skin lotion, lipstick, perfume, and eye shadow.

Beauty consultants work for companies and get paid on *commission.* This means that they keep part of the money from what they have sold. Because all companies have their own special products, they must train their own beauty consultants.

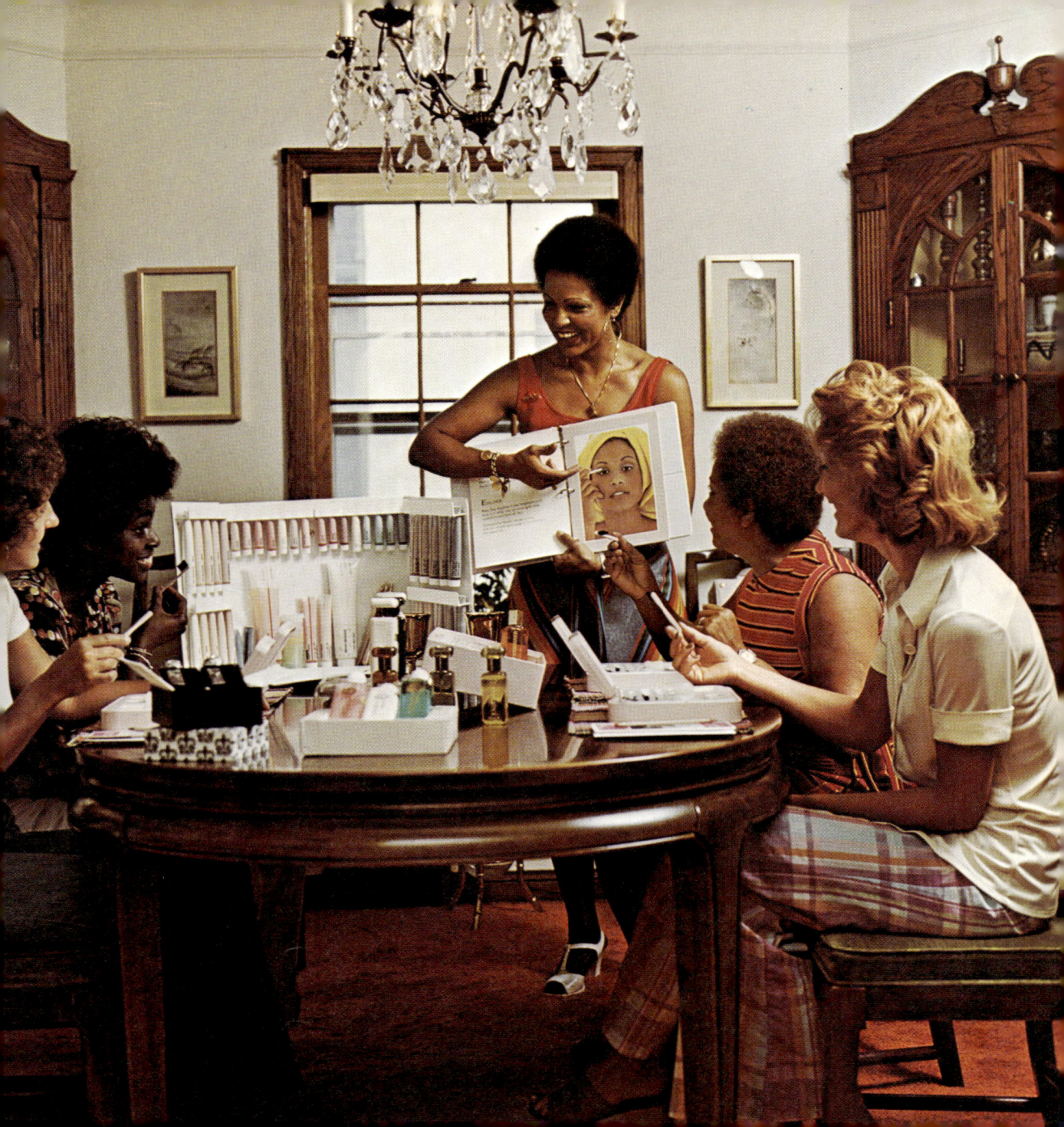

Beauty and grooming careers described in this book

Barber-Hairstylist

Beautician

Beautician's Assistant

Manicurist

Skin Care Specialist

Electrologist

Hair Replacement Specialist

Wig Stylist

Beauty School Instructor

Product Formulation Chemist

Analytical Research Chemist

Testing Salon Technician

Beauty Salon Owner

Cosmetics Salesperson

Beauty Consultant

A letter from a cosmetics company executive

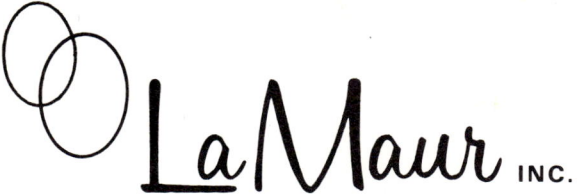

INC.

P.O. BOX 1221, MINNEAPOLIS, MINNESOTA 55440
Plant, Office and Shipping Address: 5601 East River Road, Minneapolis, Minnesota 55432

Dear Readers,

Beauty and good grooming have become an extremely important part of our American way of life.

If you would like to help people look better and feel happier, perhaps you would like a career in the field of beauty and grooming.

I hope that some of the jobs illustrated in this book will be of interest to you, and will help you to decide on a career in our growing industry.

Sincerely,

Duke Riddle
Duke Riddle
Director of Salon and
Field Product Testing

The publisher would like to thank La Maur Inc., The Barbers, Golden Plaza Coiffures, Midway College of Hair Design, Something Nice Inc., and Mrs. Hazel Tanner for their cooperation in the preparation of this book.

The photographs in this book realistically depict existing conditions in the service or industry discussed, including the number of women and minority groups currently employed.

We specialize in publishing quality books for young people. For a complete list please write

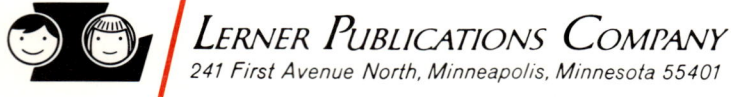

LERNER PUBLICATIONS COMPANY
241 First Avenue North, Minneapolis, Minnesota 55401

613
L   LERNER, MARK
AUTHOR
Careers in Beauty & Grooming
TITLE

DATE DUE	BORROWER'S NAME	ROOM NUMBER
MAY 21	Lea Ann Kidd	31
MAY 20	Joann Denver	34
SEP 30	Donna Mehling	43
FEB 24	Michael K	37

613
L   Lerner, Mark

Careers in Beauty & Grooming

WATERLOO LOCAL SCHOOL MIDDLE SCHOOL LIBRARY

35874